Linda Rector Page,
N.D., PhD.

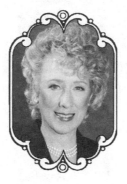

Colds & Flu
&
You

The Healthy Healing Library Series

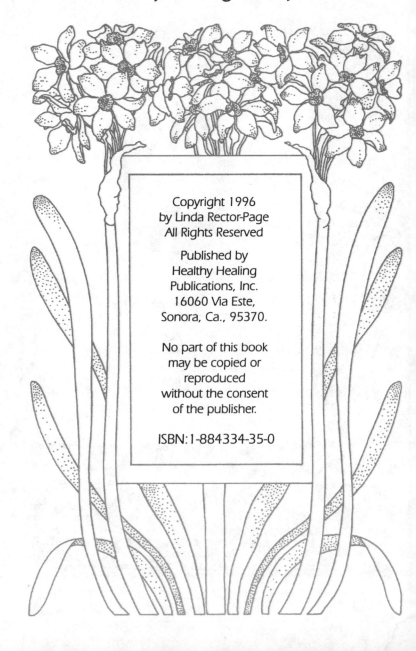

Published by
Healthy Healing
Publications, Inc.
16060 Via Este,
Sonora, Ca., 95370.

ISBN:1-884334-35-0

DR. PAGE'S WRITTEN PAPERS ARE THOROUGHLY RESEARCHED - THROUGH EMPIRICAL OBSERVATION AS WELL AS FROM INTERNATIONALLY DOCUMENTED EVIDENCE. STUDIES ARE ONGOING AND UPDATED AT HEALTHY HEALING PUBLICATIONS, 16060 VIA ESTE, SONORA, CA.,

About This Booklet

As affordable, high quality health care in America becomes more difficult to finance, access and obtain, natural therapies and healthy wellness techniques are receiving more attention.

Over 75% of Americans now use some form of natural health care, from vitamins, to cleansing diets, to massage therapy, to herbal supplements.

Everyone wants and needs more information about these methods in order to make informed choices for their own health and that of their families. The *Healthy Healing Library Series* was created to answer this need - with inexpensive, up-to-date booklets on the subjects people want to hear about the most.

The lifestyle therapy programs discussed in each booklet have been developed over the last fifteen years from the reported responses and successful healing results experienced by literally thousands of people.

In addition, the full time research team at Healthy Healing Publications, Inc. investigates herbs, herbal combinations and herbal therapies from around the world for their availability and efficacy. You can feel every confidence that the recommendations are synthesized from real people with real problems who got real results.

Herbal medicines are highlighted in the booklets because they are in the forefront of modern science today. Herbal healing has the proven value of ancient wisdom and a safety record of centuries. Yet, science can only quantify, isolate, and assay to understand. Herbs respond to these methods, but they are so much more than the sum of their parts. God shows his face a little in herbs. They, too, have an ineffable quality.

Fortunately for mankind, our bodies know how to use herbs without our brains having to know why.

Table of Contents

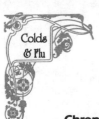

Colds & Flu & You

Chronic respiratory infections are more than common in our society today. It is estimated that at any one time, over a third of our population has had a cold or flu within the last two weeks. The national average is 2.5 colds per person per year – more than 600 million colds in alll

A "cold" is often a cleansing attempt by the body to rid itself of waste overload. Toxins and bacteria build up to a point where natural immune response cannot cope. So the wonderful, complex immune system opens up, and drains the body of excess mucous accumulation and bacterial colonies, through coughing, runny nose, sneezing or diarrhea. Then it begins to rebuild a stronger, cleaner system.

The glands are barometers of infection; since the endocrine system is on a six day cycle, a normal cold runs for about a week as the body works through its detoxification process.

> **The cleansing cure for a cold or flu infection
> is not really the problem, the cause of it is.**

Many of today's respiratory infections come from lifestyle habits that depress the immune system. Smoking, environmental pollutants, and poor diet are the most influential causes. The person who suffers frequently from sinus headaches, bronchitis, constant colds and sore throat, flu, or chronic congestion, is almost invariably one who eats a lot red meats and fatty dairy products, who likes plenty of salty, sugary, fatty foods, and is a heavy coffee drinker. Fresh fruits and vegetables are almost off this person's diet chart. A diet like this causes too much mucous to be formed in the body, and although some mucous is beneficial for membrane and tissue health, most Americans carry around 12 to 15 pounds of it. Mucous deposits become filled with toxic impurities and unreleased wastes from preservatives, chemical additives, pesticide residues, etc. They are a perfect breeding ground for harmful bacteria and virus growth.

Drugs and over-the-counter medicines only relieve the symptoms of respiratory infections. They do not cure them, and often make the situation worse by depressing immune response, drying up necessary mucous elimination, and keeping harmful bacteria, virus, or allergens, inside the body. (Yet another case of "fooling Mother Nature" that doesn't work). Anti-biotics are not effective against cold and flu virus infections. And whatever temporary relief aspirin might afford, it can enhance viral replication.

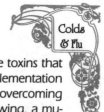

A short, liquid diet to eliminate excess mucous (and the toxins that go with it), diet improvement, outdoor exercise and supplementation with herbs are the most beneficial and quickest means of overcoming colds and flu. Herbal combinations can work with, or following, a mucous cleansing diet. They increase oxygen uptake in the lungs and tissues, encourage adrenal gland function, and allow better sleep while progress on the underlying causes is taking place.

Do You Have A Cold or The Flu?
Colds and flu respond to different treatment. Here are the differences.

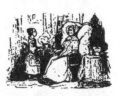

Colds and flu are distinct and separate upper respiratory infections, triggered by different viruses. (Outdoor environment, drafts, wetness, temperature changes, etc. do not cause either of these illnesses.) As previously noted, colds are a natural way for the body to cleanse itself of toxic build-up. They increase elimination by sweating and mucous discharge. This elimination makes us unusually tired so that we rest. A cold automatically activates immune response.

Most people feel much better after a cold because the body makes healing and environmental adjustments.

The flu is more serious, because it can spread to the lungs, and cause severe bronchitis or pneumonia. Initial symptoms for each condition may be similar because both colds and flu begin when viruses penetrate the body's protective barriers. Nose, eyes, and mouth are usually the sites of invasion for common cold viruses such as rhinovirus or corona virus. The most likely entry target for the flu virus is the respiratory tract.

The following brief **SYMPTOM CHART** can help identify your particular condition, so that you can choose a therapy for your needs.

A COLD PROFILE LOOKS LIKE THIS:
- Slow onset.
- No prostration.
- Rarely accompanied by fever and headache.
- Localized symptoms such as runny nose and sneezing.
- Mild fatigue and weakness from body cleansing.
- Mild to moderate chest discomfort, usually with a hacking cough.
- Sore throat common, especially at the beginning.

Colds
& Flu

A FLU PROFILE LOOKS LIKE THIS:
- •Swift, severe onset.
- •Early and prominent prostration with flushed, hot, moist skin.
- •Accompanied by high (102°-104°) fever, headache and sore eyes.
- •General symptoms of chills, depression and body aches.
- •Digestive symptoms of diarrhea and stomach soreness.
- •Extreme fatigue, sometimes lasting 2-3 weeks.
- •Acute chest discomfort, with severe hacking cough.
- •Sore throat occasionally.

❧Coping with the "common" cold naturally

With a healthy, functioning immune system, a toxin-eliminating cold should not last more than four days. For this type of minor-misery cold, increasing rest time, drinking cleansing teas, and taking a natural immune activator is all that is needed to send you on your way with a cleansed system.

An effective herbal program to pursue as soon as the first signs of a cold appear might be as follows:
- •Take 15 to 30 drops **ECHINACEA EXTRACT** (PD - 4499) twice daily, to flush the lymph glands and act as a mild antibiotic.
- •Take 4 to 6 capsules daily of a cold season defense formula.

GARLIC, ACEROLA CHERRY, BAYBERRY, ASCORBATE VIT. C, VEG. ACIDOPHILUS, BEE POLLEN, PARSLEY, GINGER RT., ROSEMARY, BONESET, ST. JOHNS WORT, ECHINACEA ANGUSTIFOLIA RT., CAPSICUM. (PD - 1900)

Note: This formula may also be used as a preventive in the very early stages.
- •Take an expectorant tea to release mucous build-up faster.

MA HUANG HERB, LICORICE RT., PLEURISY RT., MULLEIN LF., ROSE HIPS, MARSHMALLOW RT., PEPPERMINT, FENNEL SD. & OIL, BONESET HERB, GINGER RT. & OIL, CALENDULA FLR., STEVIA HERB. (B - 5930)

If your cold has gained a firm foothold, throwing it off becomes more difficult. Even so, an effective herbal program can come to your rescue. Herbs work with the body systems to reduce severity and duration of symptoms and enhance immune response. They promote perspiration and cleansing, and help you to get much needed rest.
- •A prime herbal drink, rich in vitamin C and bioflavonoids, to take for entrenched cold might look like this:

PEAR FLAKES, CRANBERRY, APPLE PECTIN, ACEROLA CHERRY, HONEY CRYSTALS, ROSE HIPS, LEMON PEEL, ORANGE PEEL, HAWTHORN BRY., HIBISCUS FLR., GINKGO BILOBA, RUTIN, BILBERRY LF. (PD - 8050)

7

Most people, especially children, experience a slight to moderate fever during a tough cold. While we know that elevated body temperature is uncomfortable, a fever is one of nature's tools for shortening the duration of an infection - especially that of a virus, **because heat deactivates virus replication.**

During a fever, body temperature is naturally raised to literally "burn out" infective poisons; to throw them off through heat and then through sweating. Unless a fever is exceptionally high, (over 103° for kids and 102° for adults) or long lasting, (more than two full days), it is usually a wise choice to let it run its natural course, even with children. Children's fevers often naturally exceed those of adults by a few degrees. Our experience is that they get better faster than if you try to suppress the fever.

If you are concerned, here are some watchwords for fevers and kids: **It's probably ok unless:**

1) you have an infant with a temperature over 100°.

2) the fever has not abated after three days, and is accompanied by vomiting, a cough and troubled breathing.

3) your child displays extreme lethargy and looks severely ill.

4) your child is making strange, twitching movements.

Administer lots of liquids during a fever - juices, water, broths, and herbal teas. Bathe frequently. Infection and toxic waste from the illness are largely thrown off through the skin. If not washed off regularly, these substances just lay on the skin and are partially re-absorbed into the body.

Toxin elimination means substantial body odor during a cleansing fever, so frequent baths and showers help you feel better, too. A cup of hot bayberry or elder flower tea, or cayenne and ginger capsules, will speed up the cleansing process by encouraging body temperature to rise and by stimulating circulation.

> **Fevers are a result of the problem and a part of the cure.**

A combination of natural therapies works best for a severe cold. Start with herbal remedies.

•During the onset and acute phase, take an herbal "first aid" formula to promote sweating and eliminate toxins. It should have plenty of naturally-occurring vitamin C and might look like this:

ASCORBATE VIT. C, BAYBERRY, GINGER RT., WHITE PINE BK., ROSE HIPS, WHITE WILLOW, CLOVES, CAPSICUM. (PD - 1950)

Note: This formula may also be used as a preventive. You might not get a bad cold after all!

8

•Take a golden seal/echinacea extract - 15 drops every 2 hours. An effective formula might look like the one below:

ECHINACEA ANGUSTIFOLIA AND PURPUREA, GOLDENSEAL RT., PAU D' ARCO, MYRRH, VEGETABLE GLYCERINE, WINTERGREEN OIL. (PD - 4678)

•Apply herbal source zinc extract drops directly on a sore throat.

ECHINACEA ANGUSTIFOLIA RT., SPIRULINA, GOTU KOLA, BARLEY GRASS, PEPPERMINT, ALFALFA , BILBERRY BRY., YELLOW DOCK RT. (PD - 4830)

Note: Zinc-providing herbs may also be used over two to three month high risk seasons to help strengthening immunity.

•Take food and plant enzymes supplements for better assimilation.

When the acute phase has passed, take an herbal combination to cleanse the lymph glands, reduce inflammation and process out harmful pathogenic wastes. A formula like the one below has the ability to address a broad spectrum of symptoms, such as swollen glands, bronchitis, throat and sinus infections. Take it for the duration of your cold symptoms, especially if your cold seems to hang on.

ECHINACEA ANGUSTIFOLIA RT., GOLDENSEAL RT., CAPSICUM, MYRRH GUM, YARROW, MARSHMALLOW RT., ECHINACEA PURPUREA., BLACK WALNUT HULLS, ELECAMPANE RT., TURMERIC RT., POTASSIUM CHL. 15MG. (PD - 1150)

> Traditional drug store cold remedies sometimes make a cold last longer. They suppress symptoms, halting natural body detoxification and balancing processes. Herbal remedies work with the body to speed recovery and reduce discomfort.

‹⊷Choose a cold remedy diet.

•Go on a liquid diet during acute stages, and take a "green drink" or vegetable broth to promote mucous elimination. Avoid refined flours, sugar, and pasteurized dairy foods. They increase production of thick mucous. When the acute stage has passed, eat light meals, including plenty of fresh and steamed vegetables, fresh fruits and juices, and cultured foods for friendly intestinal flora.

•Drink plenty of liquids; 6-8 glasses daily of fresh fruit and vegetable juices, herb teas, and water to help flush toxins out of the system.

•Eat lightly but with good nutrition. During an infection, nutrient absorption is less efficient. A vegetarian diet is the best at this time so the body won't have to work so hard at digestion.

•Take 2 TBS. cider vinegar with 2 tsp. honey in water each morning.

•Take 2 TBS. **each** lemon juice and honey, mixed with 1 teasp. fresh grated ginger at night.

☙Add essential supplements.

•Take plenty of ascorbate vitamin C or Ester C, preferably in powder form with juice, spread throughout the day: about $1/_4$ teasp. every half hour until stools are soupy, to flush the body and neutralize toxins. Begin to take vitamin C, in preventive doses of about 5000mg a day for adults at the first signs of a cold. This will shorten its length and severity and boost immune response.

•Dissolve low dose zinc lozenges under the tongue to kill pathogenic throat bacteria.

☙Slow down for a few days and get some rest.

•The value of rest and sleep cannot be over-emphasized. Immune system functions rise when the autonomic nervous system assumes control over body functions. Immune-enhancing compounds are released throughout the body during deep sleep. Most regeneration of virus-damaged cells occurs between midnight and 4 a.m. Go to bed early.

•Stay relaxed. Let the body concentrate its energy on overcoming the cold. If you exercise, take a few days off. Vigorous exercise stresses an already stressed body too much for easy recovery. However, a daily walk will rev up immune defenses and get you out of the house. A walk in fresh air puts cleansing oxygen into the lungs, and stops you from feeling sorry for yourself. It works wonders!

•Open your channels of elimination with hot baths or showers, hot broths, a little brandy and lemon, and maybe a catnip enema.

•Use a eucalyptus steam in a vaporizer to open sinus passages and quiet a cough. Increase room humidity so the mucous membranes will remain active against the virus or bacteria.

•Get a massage therapy treatment to open blocked body meridians.

•Take a hot sauna. Many toxins will pass out though the skin.

•Apply hot ginger compresses to the chest to relieve congestion.

> Think positively. Optimism is often a self-fulfilling prophecy.

☙If your cough and sore throat keep hanging on:

A hanging-on cough, sore throat or swollen glands can be the inflamed result of a severe cold, or a chronic low grade strep infection. Both of these conditions can be treated symptomatically with herbal and supplement remedies. Natural herbal medications are also excellent for children where the usual long courses of anti-biotics often do more harm than good to delicate immune defenses.

ᐖFor a chronic, low grade strep infection:

•Take 2 to 4 SHARK CARTILAGE and 6 to 8 GARLIC capsules daily.

•Use **Usnea Extract** (PD - 4992) a natural anti-biotic and anti-viral, as a throat coat; use as a gargle in water 3 times daily, or 15 drops under the tongue 2 times daily.

or

•Take vitamin C 5000mg daily and spray the throat several times daily with a grapefruit seed extract natural anti-biotic spray.

For a hanging-on cough, sore throat and swollen glands:

•Take green tea in a cleansing, anti-bacterial formula to help eliminate mucous and reduce infection. Two to three cups daily are recommended. A good green tea combination might look like this:
Bancha Lf., Kukicha Twig, Burdock Rt., Gotu Kola Herb, Fo-Ti Rt., Hawthorn Bry., Orange Peel, Cinnamon Bk. & Oil, Orange Blossom Oil. (CD - 6400)
Drop 15 drops of **Echinacea Extract** (PD - 4499) in each cup of tea for best immune-activating results.

•Suck on propolis lozenges every few hours.

•Take effervescent vitamin C several times daily. Hold in the mouth for as long as possible.

•Use a throat coat herbal tea - especially for children:
Slippery Elm Bk., Wild Cherry Bk., Licorice Rt., Fennel Sd., Orange Peel, Cinnamon Bk., Cardamom Pods, Ginger Rt., Anise Oil. (B - 5150)

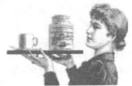

ᐖFlu infections are longer and stronger than colds.

Flu and viral respiratory infections are increasingly prevalent and insidious in America today, as air and soil pollutants, chemical foods and preservatives, and generally poor nutrition lower our immune defenses. These viruses are progressively virulent and do not respond to medical anti-biotics. Many people have been incapacitated for weeks at a time, unable to overcome them.

Flu treatment works best in stages for complete recovery.

•**For the ACUTE or INFECTIVE stage** - including aches, chills, prostration, fever, sore throat, and sometimes diarrhea, use the following remedies for 2 to 4 days.

   •Take only liquid nutrients - plenty of steamy chicken soup (yes, your grandma was right), or other hot broths to stimulate mucous release. Vegetable juices and green drinks help alkalize body chemistry and rebuild the healthy blood.

   •Take an herbal anti-viral extract several times daily. A combination of ST. JOHN'S WORT, LOMATIUM AND PROPOLIS EXTRACT (PD - 4688) is a good choice. Take 15 drops at a time under the tongue or in lemon balm tea for best results.

   •Take an herbal "crisis management" formula to raise body temperature, inhibit virus replication, and induce sweating.
ROSE HIPS AND ASCORBATE VIT. C, BAYBERRY, GINGER RT., WHITE PINE BK., WHITE WILLOW, CLOVES, CAPSICUM. (PD - 1950)

   •Take vitamin C in crystal or powder form, $1/_4$ teasp. every half hour to bowel tolerance to flush wastes fast and neutralize toxicity.

   •Get **plenty** of bed rest to revitalize your immune system.

   For the RECUPERATIVE or HEALING stage, to restore the body's natural resistance, use the following remedies for one to two weeks.

   •Follow a vegetarian, light, "green" diet. Have a salad every day, eat cultured foods like yogurt and kefir for friendly flora replacement, and steamed vegetables with brown rice for strength.

   •Take a daily green drink for vitality and rebuilding healthy blood. An effective green drink mix might look like this:
RICE PROTEIN, BARLEY GRASS & SPROUTS, ALFALFA LEAF & SPROUTS, BEE POLLEN, ACEROLA CHERRY, OAT & QUINOA SPROUTS, APPLE PECTIN, SIBERIAN GINSENG RT., SARSAPARILLA, SPIRULINA, CHLORELLA, DANDELION RT. & LF., DULSE, LICORICE RT., GOTU KOLA LF, AND APPLE JUICE. (SA - 8150)

   •Take an herbal immune activator, such as ECHINACEA EXTRACT (PD - 4499) or REISHI/GINSENG EXTRACT (PD - 4446) or use **osha root tea** for children.

   •Continue with vitamin C in capsule form - up to 5000mg daily.

   •Take food or herbal enzymes with supplements for better assimilation.

   •Use overheating therapy to overcome flu viruses. Take a hot sauna, hot spa soak, or hot bath to raise body temperature and increase circulation. Overheating therapy is a traditional therapy dating back to ancient Greek medical practice as an effective way to deactivate viruses.

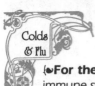

{●**For the IMMUNE SUPPORT stage**, to strengthen and stabilize the immune system especially during high risk flu season, use the remedies for this stage for two to three weeks.

●During immune-building stages, indeed all stages, avoid all refined foods, sugars, and pasteurized dairy foods. They increase mucous clogging and allow a place for the virus to live. Avoid alcohol and tobacco as immune suppressors. Avoid caffeine-containing foods. They inhibit iron and zinc absorption.

●Begin the immune support stage with a complete massage therapy treatment. It helps you to feel better right away, clears body meridians and cleanses remaining pockets of toxins.

●Take a system strengthening drink two to three times a week for a month to alkalize the body and add concentrated food source minerals. Such a drink mix might look like this:
HERBAL BLEND: ALFALFA, BORAGE SD., YELLOW DOCK RT., OATSTRAW, DANDELION, BARLEY GRASS, LICORICE RT., WATERCRESS, PAU D'ARCO, NETTLES, HORSETAIL HERB, RASPBERRY, FENNEL SD., PARSLEY, BILBERRY, SIBERIAN GINSENG RT., SCHIZANDRA, ROSEMARY, *SEA VEGETABLE BLEND:* DULSE, WAKAME, KOMBU, SEA PALM. *FOOD BLEND:* MISO, SOY, TAMARI, CRANBERRY JUICE, NUTRITIONAL YEAST. (SA - 8230)

If you still just can't seem to "get over it", make up a gallon of the following cleansing, purifying tea, and take 5 to 6 cups daily with 12 to 15 herbal colon cleansing capsules daily until the virus is removed.
The tea:
RED CLOVER , HAWTHORN, HORSETAIL, ECHINACEA PURPUREA LF., MILK THISTLE SD., PAU D'ARCO BK., GOTU KOLA HERB, LEMONGRASS & OIL, BLUE MALVA FLR., YERBA SANTA LF. (CD- 5120)
The capsules:
BUTTERNUT BK., CASCARA SAGRADA, TURKEY RHUBARB RT., PSYLLIUM HUSKS, BARBERRY BK., FENNEL SD., LICORICE RT., GINGER RT., IRISH MOSS, CAPSICUM FRUIT. (CD - 2350)

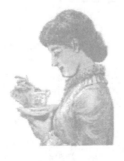

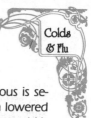

Getting Rid of Bronchitis

Chronic bronchitis is a condition in which excessive mucous is secreted in the bronchi. The typical victim is forty or older, with lowered immunity from prolonged stress, fatigue or smoking. Chronic bronchitis usually develops slowly over a series of years, **but will not go away on its own.** Slowly the bronchial walls thicken and the number of mucous-filled glands increases. The person becomes increasingly susceptible to respiratory infections, during each of which bronchial tissue becomes more inflamed, and mucous becomes thicker and more profuse.

Air pollutants are probably responsible for more chronic bronchitis than any other one cause. Avoid smoking, second-hand smoke and smog-plagued areas. Get fresh air and sunshine every day if possible.

The recent type of **viral bronchitis** which affects women is exceptionally hard to treat, and lasts from three weeks to five months. **Bacterial bronchitis** can be incapacitating and lead to serious, even potentially fatal lung disease. Get a professional diagnosis if you feel you have either bacterial or viral bronchitis.

The natural therapy treatments recommended in this section are general, for most bronchitis symptoms.

A program to overcome chronic respiratory conditions is usually more successful when begun with a short mucous elimination diet. Take cleansing vegetable juices and green drinks, high vitamin C fruit juices, broths, hot tonics, herb teas and bottled water. (See HEALTHY HEALING-*Tenth Edition* by Linda Rector-Page, for a detailed Mucous Congestion Cleanse.)

Then, follow a mainly vegetarian (green salads, vegetables and rice) diet for several weeks. Avoid or reduce fatty foods, dairy products, salts and heavy, starchy foods to lessen congestion. Drink plenty of cleansing, detoxifying liquids, such as vegetable broths and juices, herbal teas, and green drinks like **chlorella or spirulina**. (See COOKING FOR HEALTHY HEALING by Linda Rector Page for a complete non-mucous forming diet).

Avoid refined sugars during healing. New studies show that sugar reduces the ability of white blood cells to fight bacteria.

•Make an onion/honey syrup to dissolve mucous and help fight a bronchial cough: Cook 5 to 6 onions and $^1/_2$ cup honey over very low heat for two hours. Strain and take 1 TB. every two hours.

•Herbal medicines for bronchitis should contain herbs with anti-oxidant, anti-viral and anti-biotic properties, like the extract formula below. MULLEIN, GRINDELIA, USNEA BARBATA, OSHA RT., COLTSFOOT, LICORICE RT., GOLDENSEAL RT., LOBELIA, TANGERINE ESS. OIL. (B- 4720)

•Herbal expectorant teas are effective to rid the chest and lungs of infection-containing mucous. A formula for adults might look like this:
MA HUANG HERB, LICORICE RT., PLEURISY RT., MULLEIN LF., ROSE HIPS, MARSHMALLOW RT., PEPPERMINT, FENNEL SD. & OIL, BONESET HERB, GINGER RT. & OIL, CALENDULA FLR., STEVIA HERB. (B- 5930)

A bronchitis formula for children might look like this: licorice rt., horehound, lemon grass, osha, coltsfoot, lobelia, pleurisy rt., mullein. Steep in a pot with 4 cups water for 25 minutes.

or use

USNEA EXTRACT (PD- 4992), an expectorant which also has antibiotic and antiviral properties.

•Increase mucous-loosening activity:

1. Apply cayenne/ginger compresses to the chest; add 6 garlic capsules daily.

2. Use a peppermint oil or eucalyptus steam. Put 2 drops of peppermint oil into a pot of boiling water. Remove from heat and drape a towel over your head and the pot to enclose the volatile oils. Inhale the steam for 5 to 10 minutes. After the steam, apply alternating hot and cold witch hazel compresses to the chest to stimulate circulation.

3. Rub tea tree oil on the chest.

4. Take a hot sauna; follow with a brisk rubdown, and chest/back percussion with a cupped hand to loosen mucous.

•Other effective therapies for bronchitis:

•Take vitamin C crystals with bioflavonoids $1/_4$ tsp. at a time in water. Initially, take up to 10,000mg or until stool turns soupy, then reduce to 3 to 5000mg daily. Take with magnesium 800mg daily for best results.

•Take bromelain 1500mg daily as an anti-inflammatory, and for prime enzyme therapy

•Take supplemental antioxidants, such as beta carotene 100,000IU or CoQ_{10} 100 mg 2x daily.

•Do deep breathing exercises daily, morning and before bed to clear lungs. But avoid inhaling cold air. Cover mouth and nose with a scarf or mask so that infectious micro-organisms are not sucked into the lungs.

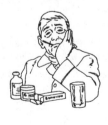

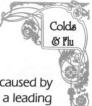

What If Your Cold Turns Into Pneumonia?

Pneumonias and pleurisy are inflammatory lung diseases caused by a wide spectrum of micro-organisms. Acute pneumonia is still a leading cause of death in America, especially among the elderly. Low immune function and immuno-suppressive drugs are common denominators that allow pneumonia to take hold. Get a professional diagnosis if you think you have pneumonia.

Bacterial pneumonia, contracted most often by children, is usually caused by staph, strep or pneumo-bacilli. It responds to anti-biotics, both medical and herbal.

Viral pneumonia, an acute systemic disease, is caused by a variety of virulent viruses, and does not respond to anti-biotics. Herbal anti-virals have shown some success.

Pleurisy, an inflammation of the pleura membrane surrounding the lungs, often accompanies pneumonia with burning sensation symptoms.

> Pneumonia is serious. No matter what kind you have it will drastically weaken your immune system. It can take 3 months to recover strength and up to 2 years to be able to resist a cold or flu without falling victim to another bout of pneumonia.

☛A diet to overcome pneumonia should be mucous-cleansing, and largely liquid for 1 to 3 days during the acute stages. Take cleansing vegetable juices and green drinks, high vitamin C fresh fruit juices, soup broths, hot tonics, herb teas and bottled water. (See *Healthy Healing-Tenth Edition* by Linda Rector Page for details on mucous congestion cleansing).
Good specifics include:
- A hot lemon and honey drink with water each morning.
- Fresh carrot juice
- A potassium juice made in your juicer for cleansing, neutralizing acids, and rebuilding the body. It consists of 3 CARROTS, 3 STALKS CELERY, ¹/₂ BUNCH SPINACH, and ¹/₂ BUNCH PARSLEY per drink, and is a blood and body purifier.

If you do not have a juicer, make a potassium broth and drink it as a soup. While not as concentrated, it is still an excellent source of energy, minerals and electrolytes. Cover with water in a large pot: 4 CARROTS, 2 POTATOES with skins, 1 ONION, 3 STALKS CELERY, ¹/₂ BUNCH PARSLEY, ¹/₂ HEAD CABBAGE, ¹/₂ BUNCH BROCCOLI. Simmer 30 minutes. Strain and discard solids. Add 2 tsp. Bragg's LIQUID AMINOS or 1 tsp. miso.

•Then follow a largely fresh foods diet for 1-2 weeks. Make sure to include plenty of vegetable protein foods like sprouts and whole grains for plant enzymes. Avoid meats, dairy products and animal fats, to allow lungs to heal easily. (For details see *Cooking For Healthy Healing* by Linda Rector Page on "Defensive Nourishment; Building Immune Power".

•Add cultured foods, such as yogurt and kefir.

•If your body keeps hanging on to a lot of congestion, try this emergency measure (not for children). Take fresh grated horseradish root in a spoon with lemon juice. Hang over a sink to immediately expel large quantities of mucous.

Infections from the viruses or microorganisms that cause pneumonia are anti-oxidant depleters, so antioxidants should be one of your therapy choices. **Herbal antioxidants** help the body take in and use oxygen better. **Antioxidant supplements** help the immune system to perform better.

Antioxidants are substances which unite with oxygen, protecting the cells and other body constituents such as enzymes from being destroyed by oxidation. Antioxidant mechanisms are very selective, acting against unwanted oxygen reactions but promoting desirable oxygen reactions.

Increasing evidence is showing that people live more vigorous, less-diseased lives when anti-oxidants are a part of their nutritional program. This is especially true if a person shows signs of immune deficiency by succumbing to frequent infections, or cannot get over an infection.

* In addition to the anti-viral or anti-bacterial herbal formulas in this booklet, **anti-oxidant herbs** should be included in a natural therapy program to overcome pneumonia. An herbal "green" drink is full of antioxidants. It also has highly absorbable, potent chlorophyllins, complex carbohydrates, complete minerals, trace minerals and proteins, and a full spectrum amino acid complex. It restores energy, increases vitality and stabilizes normal body functions. It combines high energy herbs, the building/rejuvenating qualities of rice and bee pollen, with the high-oxygen therapeutic benefits of sea and land greens. Chlorophyll is very close to human hemoglobin in composition. Taking in a green drink is like giving yourself a little transfusion for health.

RICE PROTEIN, BARLEY GRASS & SPROUTS, ALFALFA LEAF & SPROUTS, BEE POLLEN, ACEROLA CHERRY, OAT & QUINOA SPROUTS, APPLE PECTIN, SIBERIAN GINSENG RT., SARSAPARILLA, SPIRULINA, CHLORELLA, DANDELION, DULSE, LICORICE RT., GOTU KOLA, AND APPLE JUICE. (SA-8150)

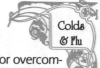

•**Bacterial pneumonia** - use an anti-bacterial formula for overcoming infections and inflammation. Look for a capsule formula such as this: ECHINACEA ANGUSTIFOLIA RT., GOLDENSEAL RT., CAPSICUM FRUIT, MYRRH GUM, YARROW, MARSHMALLOW RT., ECHINACEA PURPUREA RT. & LF., BLACK WALNUT HULLS, ELECAMPANE RT., TURMERIC RT., POTASSIUM CHLORIDE 15MG. (PD - 1150)

•**Viral pneumonia** - use an extract containing herbs that have anti-viral properties. The following combination has a long history of success against virally caused illness, even in cases where antibiotic drugs have not. ST. JOHN'S WORT, LOMATIUM AND PROPOLIS (PD - 4688) is a good choice. Take 15 drops at a time under the tongue or in lemon balm tea several times daily for best results.

•Effective anti-oxidant herbs can address symptomatic lung/chest congestion and afford breathing relief for deep-seated respiratory infections. The best effects from a "first aid" anti-oxidant formula are long term. They encourage better oxygen uptake by the body and help stimulate immune response. A good capsule combination to take during the acute stage of pneumonia might look like this:
ROSE HIPS AND ASCORBATE VIT. C, BAYBERRY, GINGER RT., WHITE PINE BK., ROSE HIPS, WHITE WILLOW, CLOVES, CAPSICUM. (PD - 1950)

•A broader based anti-oxidant formula to help heal the lungs after the crisis has passed might look like this:
MULLEIN, WILD CHERRY BK., GINKGO BILOBA, SLIPPERY ELM BK., MARSHMALLOW RT., CHICKWEED, LICORICE RT., KELP, ACEROLA CHERRY FRUIT, CINNAMON BK., MA HUANG HERB, CAPSICUM. (B - 3860)

•An herbal diuretic/anti-oxidant combination to remove excess fluid from the lungs (critical in treatment for pneumonia) might look like this:
CORNSILK, JUNIPER BERRY, UVA URSI, DANDELION ROOT, MARSHMALLOW ROOT, GOLDENSEAL ROOT, GINGER ROOT, PARSLEY ROOT & LEAF, HONEY. (CD - 4700)

•An anti-inflammatory/anti-oxidant combination to reduce pain and swelling of the lungs and chest may be taken throughout the healing process as needed, and might look like this:
WHITE WILLOW BK., ST. JOHN'S WORT, ECHINACEA ANGUSTIFOLIA RT., ECHINACEA PURPUREA RT., WHITE PINE BK., GOTU KOLA, RED CLOVER., DEVIL'S CLAW RT., ALFALFA, BURDOCK, DANDELION RT., CHAMOMILE, UVA URSI LF., GINGER RT., BROMELAIN 22MG. (CO - 1180)

•The best green source to rebuild immune response from pneumonia is chlorella extract. The best adaptogenic herb to normalize body functions after pneumonia is panax ginseng. Together, they are a powerful combination for healing. **CHLORELLA/GINSENG EXTRACT** (SA - 4442)

☙Specific supplement therapy for pneumonia should include both antioxidant and anti-inflammatory activity.
•PCOs from grape seed or white pine- 100mg 3 daily.
•CoQ$_{10}$ - 60mg 4 daily.
•Vitamin C with bioflavonoids and rutin - $1/4$ teasp. in water every half hour daily for two weeks during the acute stages; then every 2 hours for another two weeks to detoxify the tissues; then 3000mg daily for another month.
•Quercetin 2000mg with bromelain 1500mg daily.
•Germanium 150mg 2 daily.
•Carnitine 500mg 2x daily for lung protection.
•A system strengthening herb and sea vegetable broth, rich in antioxidants like marine carotenes and vitamin E, bioflavonoids and minerals daily for 1 month.
HERBAL BLEND: **ALFALFA, BORAGE SD., YELLOW DOCK RT., OATSTRAW, DANDELION, BARLEY GRASS, LICORICE RT., WATERCRESS, PAU D'ARCO, NETTLES, HORSETAIL, RED RASPBERRY, FENNEL SD., PARSLEY, BILBERRY BRY., SIBERIAN GINSENG RT., SCHIZANDRA, ROSEMARY.** *SEA VEGETABLE BLEND:* **DULSE, WAKAME, KOMBU, SEA PALM.** *FOOD BLEND:* **MISO, SOY, TAMARI, CRANBERRY JUICE, NUTRITIONAL YEAST.** (SA - 8230)

Overcoming Sinusitis

The sinuses are thin, resonating air-filled chambers in the cartilage around the nose, on both sides of the forehead, between the nasal passages and the eye sockets and in the cheekbones. When sinus openings are obstructed, mucous and sometimes infected pus collect in the sinuses causing pain and swelling. **Acute sinusitis** is an inflammation of the mucous membranes that line the sinuses. A viral cold is the most common condition for acute sinusitis. **Chronic sinusitis** often causes nasal polyps and scar tissue. Natural healing methods revolve around relieving the clog and inflammation, and neutralizing the viral infection.

Suppressive drugstore remedies can trigger a sinus infection by suppressing natural drainage of infective material, or by aggravating a current infection by driving it deeper into the sinuses.

{▶Sinusitis may be effectively addressed both symptomatically and caus-
ally with herbal therapies.

•**GOLDENSEAL ROOT** is a specific herbal remedy for sinusitis. A
dilute golden seal root tea can be used as a nasal wash. Just close one
nostril and sniff the tea up the open nostril.)

•I also recommend taking an herbal anti-biotic combination with
golden seal and echinacea to jump start the healing process. Even
though, like most people, you may not have had success with chemical
antibiotics for your sinusitis, herbal anti-biotics work differently. Instead of
trying to overwhelm the infecting organism, antibiotic herbs work to
flush the lymph glands and reduce inflammation so that the body can
process the poisons out itself. The herbs in the following capsule formula
also stimulate the immune system to strengthen the body against chronic
infection.

ECHINACEA ANGUSTIFOLIA RT., GOLDENSEAL RT., CAPSICUM FRUIT, MYRRH
GUM, YARROW, MARSHMALLOW RT., ECHINACEA PURPUREA RT. & LF., BLACK
WALNUT HULLS, ELECAMPANE RT., TURMERIC RT., POTASSIUM CHLORIDE
15MG. (PD - 1150)

•Or take USNEA EXTRACT (PD - 4992), 15 drops every 4 hours for the
first week of healing.

•A symptom-relieving formula for sinus headache, stuffiness and
watery eyes might look like this: MARSHMALLOW RT., MA HUANG, BEE
POLLEN, WHITE PINE BK., GOLDENSEAL RT., BURDOCK RT., JUNIPER BRY.,
PARSLEY RT., ACEROLA CHERRY, ROSEMARY, MULLEIN LF., CAPSICUM FRUIT,
LOBELIA HERB, PANTOTHENIC ACID 20MG, VIT B$_6$ 20MG. (B - 1200)

•A fast-acting herbal expectorant releases mucous buildup in the
head and chest. It encourages sinus pressure release through drainage,
and is gentle enough to be used by children, even when there are aller-
gies involved. It might look as follows:

MA HUANG HERB, LICORICE RT., PLEURISY RT., MULLEIN LF., ROSE
HIPS, MARSHMALLOW RT., PEPPERMINT LF., FENNEL SD. & OIL,
BONESET HERB, GINGER RT., CALENDULA, STEVIA HERB. (B - 5930)

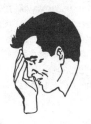

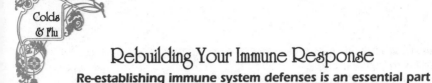

Rebuilding Your Immune Response

Re-establishing immune system defenses is an essential part of overcoming a cold or flu infection.

Maintaining strong immune defenses in today's world is not easy. Daily exposure to environmental pollutants, the emotional and excessive stresses of modern lifestyles, chemicalized foods, and new virus mutations are all a challenge to our immune systems.

Immune defense is autonomic and subconscious. It's a system that works on its own to fend off or neutralize disease toxins, and to set up a healing environment for the body. It is this quality of being a part of us, yet not under our conscious control, that is the great power of immune response. It is also the dilemma of medical scientists as they struggle to get control of a system that is all pervasive and yet, in the end, impossible to completely understand.

The immune system is not responsive to drugs for healing. In fact, an overload of antibiotics, antacids, immunizations, cortico-steroid drugs, and environmental pollutants can affect immune system balance to the point where it cannot distinguish harmful cells from healthy cells.

Three unwanted things often happen when we use too many drugs: 1) Our bodies may build up a tolerance to the drug so that it requires more of it to get the same effect. 2) The drug slowly overwhelms immune response so the body becomes dependent upon it, using it as a crutch instead of doing its own work. 3) The drug misleads the body's defense system to the point that it doesn't know what to assault, and attacks everything in confusion. This type of over-reaction often happens during an allergy attack, where the immune system may respond to substances that are not really harmful.

Even doctors admit that most drugs really just stabilize the body, or arrest a harmful organism, to allow the immune system to gather its forces and take over. The character of immune response varies widely between people, making it almost impossible to form a drug that will stimulate immunity for everyone. If we use drugs wisely to stimulate rather than over kill, if we "get out of the way" by keeping our bodies clean and well nourished, the immune system will spend its energies rebuilding instead of fighting, and strengthen us instead of constantly gathering resources to conduct a "rear guard" defense.

Natural nutritive forces, like healing foods and herbal medicines **can and do** support the immune system. They enhance its activity, strengthen it, and provide an environment through cleansing and detoxification for it to work at its best.

21

Enzyme Therapy, Herbs & Immune Response

Enzymes are basic and critical to immune response.
The very nature of immune strength means that it must be built from the inside out. Nowhere is enzyme activity more important.

☙Here's how enzyme therapy works.

Enzyme therapy uses metabolic enzymes to stimulate immune response. Metabolic enzymes are involved in every process in the body, but the link between enzymes and immunity comes from lymphocytes, or white blood cells. Immune organs, like the thymus and lymph nodes, keep a constant level of white blood cells circulating through the body to attack foreign invader cells. When toxins and foreign substances are in the body, white blood cells attack them, and break them up or digest them by secreting enzymes on their surfaces. Some diseases, like cancer, leukemia, anemia, and heart disease can even be diagnosed by measuring the amount of certain enzymes in the blood and body fluids. Chronic problems seem to respond the best to enzyme therapy. Most improvement takes place within 3 to 6 months.

As more is becoming known about enzyme deficiency identification techniques, more naturopaths are turning to plant enzyme therapy to resolve conditions from chronic digestive disorders and sore throats to hay fever, flu infections, muscle weakness, ulcers, and candida albicans. Proteolytic enzymes serve as anti-inflammatory agents for sports injuries, respiratory problems, degenerative diseases, and healing from surgery. Other enzymes clean wounds, dissolve blood clots, and control allergic reactions to drugs.

One of the most important functions of enzymes is to neutralize toxins in the body. Anti-oxidant co-enzymes, such as glutathione peroxidase, and superoxide dismutase, (SOD), scavenge and neutralize cell-damaging free radicals by turning them into stable oxygen and H_2O_2, and then into oxygen and water.

Giving your body generous, high quality plant nutrients at the first sign of infection or ill health improves your chances of destroying pathogenic bacteria. Immune-enhancing plants can be directed at "early warning" problems to build strength for immune response. Herbs and superfoods are excellent choices for enzyme therapy because they carry their own plant enzymes along with their medicinal properties. As always for the best herbal therapy effects, a combination is better, offering a wider range of enzyme activity to work with the body.

The immune system is the body system most sensitive to nutritional deficiencies. Giving your body generous, high quality, natural remedies at the first sign of infection improves your chances of overcoming a disease before it takes serious hold. Powerful, immune-enhancing superfoods and herbs can be directed at "early warning" problems to build strength for immune response. Building good immune defenses takes time and commitment, but it is worth it. **The inherited immunity and health of you, your children and your grandchildren is laid down by you.**

The respiratory problems included in this booklet, like colds, flu, bronchitis or pneumonia, respond well to enzyme therapy. Fresh fruits and vegetables are excellent sources, or get enzymes from herbal combinations that also activate the liver to obtain the most from them. The enzyme therapy formula below also helps take down the inflammation from a cold, sinus or sore throat infection.

ECHINACEA ANG. RT., SPIRULINA, GOTU KOLA, PEPPERMINT, BILBERRY, YELLOW DOCK, ALFALFA, BARLEY GRASS, PROPOLIS. (PD - 4830)

🌿Here are immune system checkpoints to keep you healthy:
✔ Add superfoods to your diet several times a week. Superfoods are a powerful way to boost immunity! Superfoods are rich in highly absorbable nutrients like chlorophyllins, enzymes, complex carbohydrates, trace minerals and a full spectrum of amino acid proteins. Superfoods include such foods as: wheat grass, barley grass, alfalfa, aloe vera, sea vegetables, microalgae, such as chlorella and spirulina, bee pollen and royal jelly. The composition of chlorophyll is very similar to that of human plasma, so these foods provide a "mini-transfusion" to detoxify your bloodstream.

An herbal "green" drink is full of superfood qualities. It restores energy, increases vitality and stabilizes normal body functions. It combines high energy "green superfood" herbs, the building/rejuvenating qualities of rice and bee pollen, with the high-oxygen therapeutic benefits of sea and land greens.

RICE PROTEIN, BARLEY GRASS & SPROUTS, ALFALFA LEAF & SPROUTS, BEE POLLEN, ACEROLA CHERRY, OAT & QUINOA SPROUTS, APPLE PECTIN, SIBERIAN GINSENG RT., SARSAPARILLA, SPIRULINA, CHLORELLA, DANDELION, DULSE, LICORICE RT., GOTU KOLA, AND APPLE JUICE. (SA - 8150)

✔ Include sea vegetables, such as kelp, dulse, kombu, wakame, and nori in your diet for their therapeutic iodine, high potassium, and sodium alginate content; or take an herbal combination like the one below, that is rich in these system-strengthening nutrients.

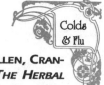

THE FOOD BLEND: YELLOW MISO, SOY PROTEIN, BEE POLLEN, CRANBERRY JUICE, NUTR. YEAST, VEGETABLE ACIDOPHILUS. *THE HERBAL BLEND*: ALFALFA, OATSTRAW, DANDELION, YELLOW DOCK RT., BORAGE SD., LICORICE RT., BARLEY GRASS, WATERCRESS, PAU D' ARCO, RASPBERRY, HORSETAIL, NETTLES, FENNEL, PARSLEY, SIB. GINSENG RT., SCHIZANDRA, BILBERRY, ROSEMARY. *SEA VEGETABLE BLEND*: SPIRULINA, DULSE, WAKAME, KOMBU, CHLORELLA, SEA PALM. (SA - 8230)

✔ Take a high potency lactobacillus or acidophilus complex, for friendly G.I. flora, and good food assimilation.

✔ Include anti-oxidants in your lifestyle, like PCOs from grapeseed and white pine, vitamin E with selenium, beta carotene, zinc, CoQ_{10}, germanium and vitamin C. Herbs with anti-oxidant qualities include echinacea, panax ginseng, reishi and maitake mushrooms, goldenseal, Siberian ginseng, licorice root, astragalus, suma and pau d' arco.

Most degenerative and chronic diseases are accompanied by free-radical damage to the immune system. The immune system membrane is crucial for immune response. The cells of the immune system are among the most susceptible to free radical damage. The membrane, or outer cell walls of the immune system have a high content of polyunsaturated fatty acids, and these fats are susceptible to oxidation.

Antioxidant enzymes help protect cell membranes, and are necessary for control of chemical sensitivities. Successful prevention of, and treatment for, most chronic infections depends on controlling dangerous free radical destruction of this cell membrane through the use of antioxidants.

•To boost antioxidants in your body, eat less fat and more fruits and vegetables, and add an herbal antioxidant supplement. An antioxidant-rich, immune support extract might look like this:
WHITE PINE BK., SIBERIAN GINSENG RT., GINKGO BILOBA, WHITE WILLOW BK., SARSAPARILLA RT., SPEARMINT, LEMON PEEL. (PD - 4780)

☙Herbal antioxidants support immune strength:
Antioxidants are vital nourishment to the control gland of the immune system - the thymus. Antioxidant-rich nutrients such as vitamin C, bioflavonoids, vitamin E, zinc, and beta carotene help prevent thymic shrinking, and encourage the activation of immune-enhancing hormones that the thymus releases.

New research shows that melatonin, an antioxidant hormone, slightly promotes thymus growth. While melatonin is not for everyone, especially people under 40, it appears to have immune-strengthening activity because of this characteristic.

Disease-resisting support herbs are rich in bioflavonoids as well as anti-oxidants for strength against free radical attacks. Key herbs also have analgesic activity. New studies indicate that many of the benefits of aspirin, such as reducing the risk of heart attack and colon cancer, are attributable to white willow, the herb from which aspirin is derived, but which does not have aspirin's gastric irritating quality.

Another is white pine bark from which pycnogenol, a prime anti-oxidant is derived. In its naturally-occurring state white pine bark has additional benefits of immune-enhancement, especially for respiratory infections. Research on both these herbs shows beneficial immune response results for the typical pneumonia symptoms of difficult breathing and shortness of breath, and they may be taken safely along with medical anti-biotics for respiratory infections.

•An antioxidant-rich, thymus stimulating formula might look like this: WHITE PINE BK., ROSEMARY, SIBERIAN GINSENG RT., GINKGO BILOBA, ASCORBATE VIT. C, ECHINACEA PURPUREA RT., ECHINACEA ANGUSTIFOLIA RT., PAU D'ARCO BK., RED CLOVER BLM., LICORICE RT., ASTRAGALUS, LEMON PEEL, LEMON BALM, GARLIC, HAWTHORN LF., FLR. & BRY., BILBERRY BRY., SPIRULINA, CAPSICUM, GINGER RT. (PD - 3840)

✔ Regular aerobic exercise keeps system oxygen high, and circulation flowing. Disease does not readily overrun a body where oxygen and organic minerals are high in the vital fluids.

✔ The immune system is stimulated by a few minutes of daily morning sunlight. But avoid excessive sun. Sun **burn** depresses immunity.

✔ Laughter lifts more than your spirits. It also boosts the immune system. Laughter decreases cortisol, an immune suppressor, allowing immune response to function better.

♦Prevention Is The Best Defense.

It is far easier to prevent a cold or flu than it is to get rid of it. This means building good health for the long run with a positive mental attitude, a healthy diet and a lifestyle as stress-free as you can make it. The newest research shows that nutritional status is the most important factor in the status of the immune system.

Herbs are holistic agents, rich in vitamins, minerals, and enzyme precursors, and are capable of becoming part of the body in a way that medicines, drugs and chemical substances are not. They are concentrated nutritional foods, and can work with the body's own enzyme activity as a source of health. This fact is the key to their success in building resistance to disease. They help repair, rebuild and restore an exhausted immune system. **I recommend two tried and true herbal formulas for cold and flu prevention. Take them during high risk seasons.**

•The following "cold season defense" capsule combination has strong anti-biotic and anti-oxidant ingredients. Taken regularly during high risk seasons, it is effective as a cold preventive. If a cold is "caught" after all, its anti-infective activity can help to shorten and soften symptoms. In a cold's acute stages, it helps throw off and neutralize toxins more quickly.
GARLIC, ACEROLA CHERRY, BAYBERRY BK., ASCORBATE VIT. C, STABILIZED VEGETABLE ACIDOPHILUS, BEE POLLEN, PARSLEY RT., GINGER RT., ROSEMARY, BONESET HERB, ST. JOHN'S WORT, ECHINACEA ANGUSTIFOLIA RT., CAPSICUM. (PD - 1900)

•An herbal anti-viral tea can address the increasing strength of today's complex infective viruses with herbs of matching complexity and strength. The following formula also has lymph-flushing herbs to clear the body of pathogens that keep your sinus infection hanging on. It may be used by children as well as adults. Take two to three cups daily during high risk seasons. For best results, take alternately for one week on and one week off, to give the body time to strengthen itself, and bring its own immune response into action.
OSHA RT., ST. JOHN'S WORT HERB, PRINCE GINSENG RT., ASTRAGALUS RT., ECHINACEA PURPUREA RT., PEPPERMINT LF. (PD - 6350)

❦

❧Herbal tonics restore and enhance immunity.
Immune building herbs are an excellent choice to revitalize the system after major illness or surgery. Ginseng, and herbs with ginseng-like qualities offer the widest range of regenerative activity. In fact, they are found in all advanced cultures around the world as sources of health restoration. Today, American ginseng species are widely respected both in this hemisphere and in the Orient for their high quality and therapeutic activity. A ginseng-rich formula for immunity might look like this:
PRINCE GINSENG RT., KIRIN GINSENG RT., ECHINACEA ANGUSTIFOLIA, PAU D'ARCO BK., SUMA RT., ASTRAGALUS RT., ECHINACEA PURPUREA RT., ST. JOHN'S WORT LF., ARALIA RT., ASHWAGANDHA RT. & LF., CHINESE WHITE GINSENG RT., SIBERIAN GINSENG RT., REISHI MUSHROOM, FENNEL SD., TIENCHI GINSENG RT., GINGER OIL. (PD - 6380)

❦

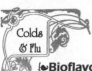

❧Bioflavonoids from herbs are key support factors you can use to maintain optimum immune response:

Herbal drink mixes are potent, unique, all natural means of delivering optimum absorption of nutrients. An herbal bioflavonoid drink is rich in naturally-occurring C complex, vitamin A, fiber and rutin. Bioflavonoids increase the effectiveness and usable levels of vitamin C, and act as direct anti-inflammatory and anti-viral agents. They stabilize the body's collagen matrix by preventing free-radical damage. Rapid therapeutic results have been reported in clearing upper respiratory symptoms.

PEAR FLAKES, CRANBERRY, APPLE PECTIN, ACEROLA CHERRY, HONEY CRYSTALS, ROSE HIPS, LEMON PEEL, ORANGE PEEL, HAWTHORN BRY., HIBISCUS FLR., GINKGO BILOBA LF., RUTIN, BILBERRY. (PD - 8050)

❧

Tonic herb compounds are best used after the acute stages of a problem to re-establish normal system functions and increase physical energy. The capsule combination below is rich in herbal anti-oxidants, providing usable tissue oxygen for increased immune strength, mental clarity and a feeling of well-being.

BEE POLLEN, SIBERIAN GINSENG RT., GOTU KOLA, SARSAPARILLA, LICORICE, SUMA, SCHIZANDRA, RICE PROTEIN PWD., ALFALFA, WILD CHERRY, BLACK COHOSH, KELP, GOLDENSEAL RT., HAWTHORN, AMERICAN PANAX GINSENG, SPIRULINA, BARLEY GRASS, GINKGO BILOBA LF., CAPSICUM, NUTR. YEAST, CHOLINE 10MG, ZINC 3MG. (E - 2250)

•A tonic tea is delicious, and may be used on a daily basis for pleasure as well as immune health and energy.

RED CLOVER, ALFALFA, HAWTHORN LF., FLR. & BRY., PRINCE GINSENG RT., SPEARMINT, DANDELION RT., WHITE SAGE, LEMONGRASS, DULSE, LICORICE, STEVIA (E - 5330)

❧

❧Put herbs on your immune defense team.

Herbal formulas have a long, world-wide history of health maintenance and disease prevention that can strengthen your stand against illness. Combinations of complementary herbs are by far the best way to take them for immune enhancement. Some effective compounds using immune enhancing herbs are detailed below:

•An "herbal defense team" tea: **RED CLOVER, HAWTHORN LF., FLR. & BRY., BURDOCK RT., LICORICE RT., SUMA RT., SCHIZANDRA BRY., ASTRAGALUS RT., WHITE SAGE, ARALIA RT., LEMONGRASS & OIL, MARSHMALLOW RT., BONESET, ST. JOHNS WORT.** (PD - 5540)

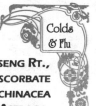

•An "herbal defense team" capsule formula: **SIBERIAN GINSENG RT., BEE POLLEN, PAU D'ARCO BK., GARLIC, BAYBERRY BK., ASCORBATE VIT. C, HAWTHORN LF., FLR. & BRY., BURDOCK RT., ECHINACEA ANGUSTIFOLIA RT., BARLEY GRASS, SUMA RT., ALFALFA LF., ASTRAGALUS RT., SCHIZANDRA BRY., GOLDENSEAL RT., RED SAGE LF., ELECAMPANE RT., KELP, YARROW FLR., ACEROLA CHERRY FRUIT, CAPSICUM FRUIT, DANDELION RT., ZINC GLUCONATE 3MG.** (PD - 2550)

•An "herbal defense team" extract formula: **GARLIC, ECHINACEA ANGUSTIFOLIA RT., SIBERIAN GINSENG RT., ROSE HIPS, HAWTHORN LF. & BRY., GOLDENSEAL RT., GUGGUL, PAU D'ARCO BK., ASTRAGALUS RT., ELECAMPANE RT., HONEY, AND PEPPERMINT OIL.** (PD - 4780)

•An herbal antioxidant capsule formula: **WHITE PINE BK., ROSEMARY, SIBERIAN GINSENG RT., GINKGO BILOBA, ASCORBATE VIT. C, ECHINACEA ANGUSTIFOLIA RT., ECHINACEA PURP. RT., PAU D'ARCO, RED CLOVER, LICORICE RT., ASTRAGALUS, LEMON PEEL, LEMON BALM, GARLIC, HAWTHORN LF., FLR. & BRY., BILBERRY, SPIRULINA, CAPSICUM, GINGER.** (PD - 3840)

New research into traditional herbal medicines for colds and flu from other healing traditions is reaching America today, offering even more validated herbal choices. Here are two of the most successful.

Green Tea & Health Maintenance

Only recently is the western healing world discovering the wonderful benefits of green tea for immunity and long term health. Studies show green tea is a potent antioxidant, scavenging free radicals better than either vitamins C or E.

Green tea is is also used as a broncho-dilator with anti-oxidant and anti-allergen flavonoids that help keep flu viruses under control. Even at "concentrations as low as one part per million, epigalocatechin gallate, a polyphenol in green tea, keeps flu viruses in check. Polyphenols in an ordinary cup of tea are 1,000 times more concentrated than this.

Green tea has potent antibacterial qualities. An herbal tea combination that takes advantage of green tea's cleansing and detoxifying benefits might look like this:

Bancha Lf., Kukicha Twig, Burdock Rt., Gotu Kola Herb, Fo-Ti Rt., Hawthorn Bry., Orange Peel, Cinnamon Bk. & Oil, Orange Blossom Oil. (CD - 6400)

Aromatherapy is a sophisticated, medicinal practice which uses the power of aroma to trigger specific responses in the body. It affects both emotional and physical health, and is especially effective for respiratory conditions such as colds and flu. Inhaling the fragrance of certain essential oils can help clear the sinuses or free congestion in the chest.

Essential oils, 75 to 100 times more concentrated than dried herbs and flowers, are at the heart of aromatherapy. During the life of the plant, essential oils deliver messages through the plant structure to regulate its functions, trigger immune response to environmental stress, protect it from harm and attract insects for pollination and propagation. In essence, aromatherapy oils act in plants much like hormones do in humans. They are some of the most potent of all herbal medicines.

Aromatherapy oils aren't really oils, but distilled condensations, formed by rushing steam through plant material. The resulting fluids are volatile, non-oily, highly active essences that may be taken in by inhalation, steams, infusers, or applied topically in massages, compresses or baths. During high risk seasons, it is wise to vaporize with essential oils to help prevent the spread of bacteria and viruses through the home.

•Use eucalyptus oil in a respirator or a bath to ease symptoms. A blend of eucalyptus, fir and pine can help open up nasal passages.

•Use wintergreen to relieve lung and nasal congestion.

•Use lavender oil to help lower a fever.

•Use tea tree oil to prevent the spread of viruses and bacteria.

•Use lemon, clove, eucalyptus, pine, cinnamon, rosemary and thyme, for antiseptic activity, especially in a diffuser to keep harmful bacteria count down. They are effective for upper respiratory infections, colds and flu. Use about 30 to 50 drops oils, and let your diffuser run for 30 minutes twice a day.

•Apply eucalyptus and tea tree topically to the throat for a sore throat.

•Make a vapor rub for chest congestion, using 50 drops eucalyptus, 15 drops peppermint, and 10 drops wintergreen to 1 oz. vegetable oil. Rub into chest for relief.

•Make an analgesic rub for sore joints and muscles. Use 20 drops each of clove, eucalyptus, tea tree, and wintergreen oils in 1 oz. vegetable oil. Rub into affected area, or add $1/4$ oz. to a bath.

Bibliography & Other Reading

Alstat, E.K. *Complementary Med.* May/June (1987).

Bassett, I.B., et al. *The Medical Journal of Australia.*1990

Brinker, Francis, N.D. The Chaparral Handbook.1990

Cabrera, Chancghal. "Ginkgo and Memory Loss", Medical Herbalism. 1993

Davis, Brent W., D.C. 'New' World Class Herb, Proceedings of the Summer Meeting of the I.C.A.K. Vol. I. 1992-93

Duke, James A. *CRC Handbook of Medicinal Herbs.* 1985.

Felter, Harvey, M.D. and J. Lloyd, Phr. M., Ph.D. *King's American Dispensatory.* 1983.

Hobbs, Christopher. *Echinacea. The Immune Herb.* 1990.

Lesnau, A., et al. "Antiviral Activity of Berberine" , Pharmazie. 1990

McCaleb, Rob. "Astragalus for Immunity", Better Nutr. May 1993

Murray, Michael T., N.D. "How to Prevent the Common Cold", Health Counselor. Vol. 5, No. 1

Pizzorno, Joseph E. "Supercharge Your Immune System", Natural Health, 1994.
Rector-Page, Linda, N.D., Ph.D. Healthy Healing 10th Edition, 1996

Schoneberger, D. *Forum Immunologie.* 1992

Stansbury, Jill, N.D. "Expectorating Botanicals", Medical Herbalism.1993

Willard, Terry, Ph.D. *Reishi Mushroom: Herb of Spiritual Potency and Medical Wonder.* 1991

About the Author....

Linda Rector-Page has been working in the fields of nutrition and herbal medicine both professionally and as a personal lifestyle choice, since the early seventies. She is a certified Doctor of Naturopathy and Ph.D., with extensive experience in formulating and testing herbal combinations. She received a Doctorate of Naturopathy from the Clayton School of Holistic Healing in 1988, and a Ph.D. in Nutritional Therapy from the American Holistic College of Nutrition in 1989. She is a member of both the American and California Naturopathic Medical Associations.

Linda opened and operated the "Rainbow Kitchen," a natural foods restaurant, then became a working partner in The Country Store Natural Foods store. She has written four successful books and a Library Series of specialty books in the nutritional healing field. Today, she lectures around the country and in the media on a wide range of natural healing topics.

Linda is the founder and formulator of Crystal Star Herbal Nutrition, a manufacturer of over 250 premier herbal compounds. A major, cutting edge influence in the herbal medicine field, Crystal Star Herbal Nutrition products are carried by over twenty-five hundred natural food stores in the U.S. and around the world.

Continuous research in all aspects of the alternative healing world has been the cornerstone of success for her reference work Healthy Healing now in its tenth edition. Feedback from all these sources provides up-to-the-minute contact with the needs, desires and results being encountered by people taking more responsibility for their own health. Much of the lifestyle information and empirical observation detailed in her books comes from this direct experience.

Cooking For Healthy Healing, now in its second revised edition, is a companion to Healthy Healing. It draws on both the recipes from the Rainbow Kitchen and the more defined, lifestyle diets that she has developed for healing since then. The book contains thirty-three diet programs, and over 900 healthy recipes.

In How To be Your Own Herbal Pharmacist, Linda addresses the rising appeal of herbs and herbal healing in America. This book is designed for those wishing to take more definitive responsibility for their health through individually developed herbal combinations.

Linda's newest work is a party reference book called Party Lights, written with restaurateur and chef Doug Vanderberg. Party Lights, takes healthy cooking one step further by adding in the fun to a good diet.

Published by Healthy Healing Publications, 1996.